This book is dedicated to every who supported me during my journey into includes all of my teachers from secondary school and college.

I would also like to thank everyone who believed in me and even the people who did not believe in me as they gave me a reason prove them wrong.

Lastly, I would like to thank the one person who believed in me when I wanted to write this book.

Introduction ............................................. 1

PART I: From Student to Med Student .............. 3

Chapter One: Picking your A-Level Subjects ....... 4

Chapter Two: Work Experience ....................... 7

Chapter Three: UCAT and BMAT .................... 9

Chapter Four: Your Personal Statement ............. 18

Chapter Five: Interview Tips ........................... 22

Chapter Six: Exam Preparation ....................... 28

PART II: From Med Student to Doctor ............... 36

Chapter Seven: The Reality of Med School .......... 37

Chapter Eight: Surviving Your First Year ............ 39

About the Author .........................................41

# GET INTO MED SCHOOL AND SURVIVE: A PRACTICAL GUIDE (UK)

A Concise 3-in-1 Guide on Smashing Your A-Levels, Getting into Medical School and Advice for New Medical Students.

By

*Ahmed Ali*

© Copyright (2020) by (Ahmed Ali) - All rights reserved.

It is not legal to reproduce, duplicate, or transmit any part of this document in either electronic means or printed format. Recording of this publication is strictly prohibited.

# *Introduction*

Thank you for purchasing this book!

So, you want to become a doctor? You have come to the right place. I will be helping you on your journey to med school. And once you get into med school, I will be giving some tips that helped me survive my first year. When writing this book, I remembered the thousands of students from underprivileged families who want to become doctors and students who were not at the top of their class – like me. I wasn't the smartest kid nor was I the laziest. I did not come from a rich family of doctors. I was just a poor kid who wanted to go to university. I didn't want to study medicine until I was almost 17 so it's never too late. On my journey, I came across many books and guides on getting into med school. There were also many paid courses that "guaranteed" you a medicine offer. However, all of them were intended for elite kids who had aced their GCSE's and could afford to spend hundreds of pounds. I wasn't one of them. In fact, no one in my family had been to university and I certainly could not afford to spend a lot of money on a course. So why am I writing a book? Because I was sick of seeing aspiring medics get taken advantage of with these "crash courses". Companies charging £50 to check your personal statement is absurd and they are in it for the profit. I want to help aspiring medics achieve their dream without breaking the bank. Despite the odds being against me, I still got into med school. I have taught plenty of students and helped them get into med school. This is for the students who want to become the doctors of tomorrow but feel disadvantaged because of their grades or their financial situation. Believe in yourself. You do not need hundreds of £s to spare or an IQ of 150. Doctors aren't robots who are just book smart. They need to be hard-working, empathetic, friendly and a lot more.

Anything I mention in this book about myself is not for bragging. I have only mentioned it to motivate *you* into becoming the best version of yourself. If *I* can do it then so can you.

With that being said, anyone who wants to get into med school can benefit from this book. This e-book isn't just for those who are underprivileged. There is no sugar-coating in this book. I will tell you what you need to know. The information I provide will hopefully build your confidence and give you the tools you need to stand out from the thousands of people who are also applying. If you find any of this useful, please share this book with anyone who may benefit from it.

That's enough from me. Read this book and go fulfil your destiny.

# PART I: From Student to Med Student

I won't lie. Getting into med school is not easy – it's competitive. It will take time, effort and dedication so make sure it is the right thing for you. Stick around and I'll go through some of the realities of med school and things you should expect.

Part I of this book covers the journey from the beginning of college or sixth form to your actual A-Level examinations. I will be giving tips on what subjects to pick, work experience, UCAT/BMAT tips, personal statement tips and how to ace your A-Level exams.

Not sure if medicine is for you? Ask around! Ask med students what it's like studying medicine. Furthermore, make sure you are aware of the commitments of being a doctor. Night shifts, 12-hour shifts and looking at well…erm.. unpleasant things. Medicine is not just a simple 5-year course. It is a lifetime commitment.

Here are some statistics on med school applications from 2007 to 2014. The numbers may be slightly different now but don't let this put you off.

| Pre-Clinical Medicine (A1) UCAS application and acceptances statistics 2007 - 2014 |||||||
| Cycle Year* | Applications** | Acceptances*** | Ratio of applications per 10 acceptances (rounded up to nearest whole number) | Percentage of applications being accepted | Percentage of applications accepted relative to 2007 |
| --- | --- | --- | --- | --- | --- |
| 2007 | 72,275 | 7,305 | 99:10 | 10.1% | 100.0% |
| 2008 | 69,020 | 7,560 | 92:10 | 11.0% | 103.5% |
| 2009 | 69,865 | 7,520 | 93:10 | 10.8% | 102.9% |
| 2010 | 80,060 | 7,530 | 107:10 | 9.4% | 103.1% |
| 2011 | 83,185 | 7,325 | 114:10 | 8.8% | 100.3% |
| 2012 | 81,260 | 7,150 | 114:10 | 8.8% | 97.9% |
| 2013 | 82,440 | 6,805 | 122:10 | 8.3% | 93.2% |
| 2014 | 84,850 | 6,820 | 125:10 | 8.0% | 93.4% |

# Chapter One: Picking Your A-Level Subjects

Your journey begins here. You've completed your GCSE's and now it's time to pick your A-Level subjects. I'm not going to sit here and sugar-coat it by saying you can study medicine by doing any subjects at A-Level. You want your application to be as competitive as possible. Whilst doing four subjects looks good, it means nothing if the grades you get aren't all A's. Therefore, I would recommend doing three unless you are confident that you can manage your time efficiently across all four subjects. I would strongly recommend picking Chemistry, Biology and Maths (or Physics). This will not only strengthen your application, but also keep all medical schools open to you. Not picking Maths or Physics is not the end of the world but some medical schools may not accept it – keep this in mind. I suggest going through the entry requirements of the universities that appeal to you the most. You *can* get away with doing Biology, Chemistry and an A-Level you enjoy (as long as you can achieve a grade A) to keep most med schools open to you.

**Why These Subjects?**

They equip you with the right skills to succeed in med school. The first few months of med school is like A-Level Biology on steroids. It is quite tough and takes some time to adapt to. However, studying Biology gives you basic background knowledge when it comes to things like neurology and cardiology.

Chemistry helps with topics like pharmacology. Knowing about intermolecular forces and a bit about organic chemistry helps in medicine.

How about Maths? It helps with problem-solving. Maths forces you to think about different ways to arrive at the same answer. As a doctor, you'll be required to solve problems and think outside the box.

Most importantly, these subjects are required by med schools. Love them or hate them, becoming a doctor without them is super hard.

I have included some typical questions you can expect in your exams for biology, chemistry and maths respectively. In the next chapter, we will be going through what is required for your medical work experience.

---

0 1 . 1  When a nerve impulse arrives at a synapse, it causes the release of neurotransmitter from vesicles in the presynaptic knob.

Describe how.

[3 marks]

---

A biology question taken from an AQA paper.

**01** Iodide ions are oxidised to iodine by hydrogen peroxide in acidic conditions.

$$H_2O_2(aq) + 2H^+(aq) + 2I^-(aq) \rightarrow I_2(aq) + 2H_2O(l)$$

The rate equation for this reaction can be written as

$$rate = k[H_2O_2]^a[I^-]^b[H^+]^c$$

In an experiment to determine the order with respect to $H^+(aq)$, a reaction mixture is made containing $H^+(aq)$ with a concentration of 0.500 mol dm$^{-3}$

A large excess of both $H_2O_2$ and $I^-$ is used in this reaction mixture so that the rate equation can be simplified to

$$rate = k_1[H^+]^c$$

**01.1** Explain why the use of a large excess of $H_2O_2$ and $I^-$ means that the rate of reaction at a fixed temperature depends only on the concentration of $H^+(aq)$.

[2 marks]

A chemistry question taken from an AQA paper.

4. (a) Write $5\cos\theta - 2\sin\theta$ in the form $R\cos(\theta + \alpha)$, where $R$ and $\alpha$ are constants, $R > 0$ and $0 \leqslant \alpha < \dfrac{\pi}{2}$

Give the exact value of $R$ and give the value of $\alpha$ in radians to 3 decimal places.

(3)

(b) Show that the equation

$$5\cot 2x - 3\operatorname{cosec} 2x = 2$$

can be rewritten in the form

$$5\cos 2x - 2\sin 2x = c$$

where $c$ is a positive constant to be determined.

(2)

A typical maths question taken from an Edexcel paper.

# Chapter Two: Work Experience

Work experience: the biggest part of your UCAS personal statement (more about that later). It is extremely important that you complete at least 3 or 4 things for your work experience. Now I appreciate that it is not easy to shadow a surgeon unless you have amazing contacts, but there are other ways to stand out. I highly recommend you get all of your work experience out of the way before you start your second year of college. The summer after your GCSE's, winter holidays, Easter holidays, half term breaks and the summer before A2 are great for work experience. This just makes you worry about one less thing during A2. Furthermore, the deadline for medical school applications is mid-October during A2 so make sure it's all done by then. The key thing to remember is that med schools look at what you have learnt from your experience and not where you did it. They want you to have a realistic idea of what it's like to be a doctor. They want you to appreciate the sacrifices and commitments that doctors make. Here are some places you can gain valuable experience from.

## GP Practice/ Hospital

This is the most obvious one. Shadowing a doctor is a great way to gain a realistic view of what their job involves. However, the main thing is what you have learned from this experience. In your personal statement, mention a particular example of teamwork and communication you saw between the multi-disciplinary team or between a doctor and patient. Always give examples. And always mention what you learned from seeing this. Do not just blab on about everything that happened as if you're telling a story. Make everything you say meaningful. Speak to doctors and patients on your placement and mention how it has improved your communication skills. Always mention how it has impacted you and what you learned from it. It's not easy getting work experience like this so email doctors and hospitals and be patient! Even if you don't manage to get work experience in a hospital it is *not* the end of the world. I would recommend contacting your local GP Practice if you cannot find any hospital placement. I appreciate that it is difficult to find a hospital placement without having the right family links.

## Care Home

This may not be the first thing that comes to mind. However, volunteering in a care home can equip you with skills that would help you during med school. Simply call or email a local care home and ask if they're willing to have someone help them out. You will have a chance to speak to some of the residents there which can improve your communication skills – mention that. You do not have to volunteer for a long time. However, if you do it long term you can mention that on your personal statement, and this will show commitment.

## Charity

Volunteering for charity is a great way to develop your communication and teamwork skills. You may be working with others but most importantly you will be helping others. This is definitely something you can mention in your personal statement especially if you have been doing it for a long time.

# Chapter Three: UCAT and BMAT

The UCAT and BMAT exams are difficult. Depending on which universities you apply to you may be required to complete one or both of them. Be sure to check the entry requirements for the four medical schools you apply to.

## **UCAT**

It was known as the UKCAT back in my day (not very long ago) but still has the same structure. Universities that require the UCAT include Aberdeen, Anglia Ruskin, Aston, Birmingham, Bristol, Cardiff, Dundee, East Anglia, Edge Hill, Edinburgh, Exeter, Glasgow, Hull York Medical School, Keele, Kent & Medway Medical School, King's College London, Leicester, Liverpool, Manchester, Newcastle, Nottingham, Plymouth, Queen Mary-University of London, Queen's University Belfast, Sheffield, Southampton, Sunderland, St. Andrew's, St. George's London and Warwick (grad only).

Start preparing for this monstrosity early. Because it *can* be tough. Start by practising questions without timing yourself to ensure accuracy. As you practice more, begin timing yourself. Be sure to book your test as soon as you finish your AS exams. This gives you a deadline to work towards. Do not pay hundreds for a UCAT crash course. I would recommend a Medify subscription for access to more than 10,000 questions. I understand it may be a bit pricey for a student, but it really is an amazing resource – it also eliminates the need to buy a UCAT book. Ask your college if they are willing to purchase subscriptions for students who are taking the UCAT. Below are the different categories you will be tested on:

| Section | Questions | Timing | Scoring |
|---|---|---|---|
| Verbal Reasoning | 44 | 22 minutes | 300-900 |
| Decision Making | 29 | 32 minutes | 300-900 |
| Quantitative Reasoning | 36 | 25 minutes | 300-900 |
| Abstract Reasoning | 55 | 14 minutes | 300-900 |
| Situational Judgement | 69 | 27 minutes | Band 1-4 |

An image taken from The Medic Portal.

The average score differs every year. However, 700+ is amazing, 650+ is solid and 600+ is okay enough for a med school to consider you if the other aspects of your application are solid. As harsh as it sounds, a score below 600 will significantly decrease your chance of being called for an interview. Let's analyse each section and go through some tips and tricks.

## **Verbal Reasoning**

In my opinion, the most difficult section. You will end up doing a lot of guessing (more about that later). You will have to read a large chunk of text and answer questions about the information given to you within the text. Practice reading quickly. Skim the text. And know the difference between true and false. True means this information was *given* to you in the text. If something was not mentioned in the text, then it is false. Never assume. Furthermore, *always* read the question before you answer it. It is tempting to skip straight to answering to save time but trust me, you'll wish you hadn't. Lastly, it is almost impossible to finish every question without guessing so go with your instinct. Make educated guesses and do not worry if you don't do too well in this section as you can make up for it in another. However, you should still aim for a solid score in every section.

### Decision Making

This section consists of multiple-choice questions and Yes/No statements. Not much can be said about this section because you either got it or you don't. Get familiar with analysing graphs quickly and analysing information as you read it. The better you are at reading and interpreting, the better you will score here. Lastly, do not overthink. Some questions are as easy as they seem whilst others may be slightly more difficult. It is important to know which questions need more time than others. Only practice with help you get better.

### Quantitative Reasoning

Many people find this section the easiest. The hardest part is using the horrible on-screen calculator. It is very time-consuming to use so get some practice using a virtual calculator. Read the questions carefully and brush up on your basic maths. Know how to work out averages such as mean, mode and median and know how to interpret charts and graphs.

### Abstract Reasoning

This section first seems impossible. With practice, it makes more sense. It will take days or even weeks to become good at this section. Start by doing these questions on Medify without timing yourself. As you get better, aim to finish them in under 25 seconds. Ask yourself if there are colour patterns, number patterns, shape patterns or ratio and symmetry. Once you establish a pattern, the rest is a cakewalk.

### Situational Judgement

This part isn't too difficult. The score for this isn't measured with a number. You'll be placed in a band from 1 to 4 – 1 being the best. This one requires you to think like a doctor. Don't answer with what *you* think is the most appropriate response. What course of action would benefit the patient or your colleague the most? I would highly recommend reading Good Medical Practice. This would give you knowledge that can not only be applied in the situational judgement test, but also in real life once you become a doctor.

Now let's talk about guessing. When should you guess answers in the UCAT? When you have 30-60 seconds remaining in a section. If you cannot make an educated guess for the remaining questions, then guess them all. You will not lose any marks and may even gain some marks. The way to guess is to pick the *same* answer for every remaining question. For example, if you have 12 questions left, guess B for all of them.

## BMAT

The BMAT exam is different to the UCAT. If you find yourself unlucky enough to do both the BMAT and UCAT, you will have to prepare wisely. Universities requiring the BMAT include the University of Oxford, University of Leeds, University of Cambridge, University College London, Lancaster University, Imperial College London and Brighton and Sussex Medical School. There are two possible dates this exam can be taken on – you cannot choose a random date like the UCAT. These include a date in September or November. There are pros and cons of taking the exam in either month. However, only the University of Oxford will **not** accept the September BMAT. I would recommend the September date because you will receive your results before the UCAS submission deadline. This allows you to change your university choices depending on how well you did on the BMAT. You will receive the November results only after submitting your application so if you didn't do too well then you may have wasted an application on a BMAT university when you should have picked a UCAT university. Also, you can only do the exam on one of these dates. You **cannot** do both.

So, let's get into the structure of the BMAT exam. It's a two-hour pen and paper exam. It is possible to take the exam at your college (speak to your college for more information). It is split into section 1 (1 hour), section 2 (30 mins) and section 3 (30 mins). Here is a table which goes into more detail about the BMAT.

| BMAT Section | What does it test? | Question format | Timing |
| --- | --- | --- | --- |
| Section 1 | Generic skills in problem solving, understanding arguments, and data analysis and inference. | 35 multiple-choice questions | 60 minutes |
| Section 2 | The ability to apply scientific knowledge typically covered in school Science and Mathematics by the age of 16 (for example, GCSE in the UK and IGCSE internationally). | 27 multiple-choice questions | 30 minutes |
| Section 3 | The ability to select, develop and organise ideas, and to communicate them in writing, concisely and effectively. | One writing task from a choice of three questions | 30 minutes |

Table taken from The Medic Portal.

Your score will be calculated, and you should receive your results in the same month you took your exam in. For section 1 and 2, a score of 5 is average, 6 is very good and 7 is exceptional. For grading information on section 3, read on ahead.

## **Section 1**

This section tests you on your problem solving and data analysis. It is somewhat similar to some aspects of the UCAT exam so it shouldn't be too difficult to grasp the basic concepts. The best way to prepare for this section is to practice without timing yourself. As you do more questions, start timing yourself and eventually aim to finish each question in less than two minutes. Always read the question before answering. Here is a typical question you can expect in section 1. BMAT Ninja is a good resource for practicing questions. The free version includes 1400+ questions and past papers. There is a paid upgrade available should you need it.

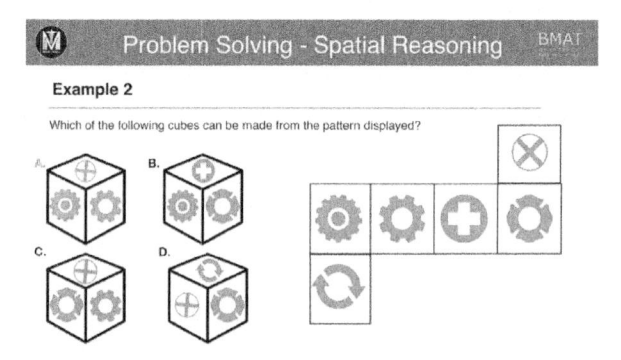

Top secret tip: take a white cube-shaped pencil eraser (a clean one) into the exam with you. When you come across a spatial awareness question like the one above, draw out the shapes accordingly onto the cube eraser. The question then becomes very easy as you can angle the eraser and see which answer is correct. No, it's not cheating and yes, it works.

## Section 2

This section *apparently* tests you on your GCSE science knowledge. I say *apparently* because many people would agree with me when I say it is much more difficult than your GCSEs. If you picked the A-Level subjects I suggested earlier on, then you will probably realise that your physics knowledge is somewhat weak at this stage. Revise it. Do not ignore physics or it will haunt you after the exam. Get some friends who do A-Level physics to go over a few things with you. Honestly, if you stay on top of your chemistry, biology and maths A-Levels then you don't have a lot to do for section 2. You will already have the required knowledge. All you need to do now is practice as many questions as you can. Here is a typical section 2 question you can expect.

> During a period of exercise, an animal inspires 120 litres of air over the course of 6 minutes. The air leaving the animal's lungs was tested to be 16% oxygen. At rest, the same animal takes in 15 litres of air per minute, which is atmospheric air at 21% oxygen. What is the rough change percentage in the volume of oxygen absorbed by the animal whilst exercising compared to at rest?
>
> A) No change.
> B) An increase $\geq 10\%$.
> C) A decrease $\geq 10\%$.
> D) An increase $\leq 10\%$.
> E) Can't tell.

## Section 3

Ah, section 3. A science student's nightmare: essays. Don't worry, this essay does not require you to analyse poems. You will be presented with three questions. You only have to answer **one** of these questions. You will get one A4 sized lined page to answer the questions – so it's not too much writing to be fair. The grade is split into two parts. You will receive a number 1 – 5 (5 being the best) to indicate the quality of the content and a letter (A, C or E) to indicate the quality of your English.

**Section 3: Written English (scored A, C or E)**

- Band A: Good use of English – clear, fluent, good use of grammar and vocabulary
- Band C: Reasonably clear use of English – reasonably fluent, some errors
- Band E: Rather weak use of English – not easy to follow, faulty grammar

**Section 3: Quality of Content (scored from 1 to 5)**

- Score 1: the essay has some bearing on the question but does not address it fully
- Score 2: addresses most of the question, but has significant elements of confusion
- Score 3: reasonably well-argued, may have weakness in the argument
- Score 4: good answer with few weaknesses, all aspects of the question are addressed
- Score 5: excellent answer with no significant weaknesses

You obviously want to aim for the highest grade possible. However, you must get at least a 3 in quality of content to have a competitive application. Brush up on your spelling, grammar and punctuation to ensure an A in written English. If you can't spell a word just don't use it – find another one. In order to get at least a 3 in quality of content, you **must** answer every part of the question. The question you choose will have multiple questions within it. Answer each one in using a clear structure and without repetition. Answer every part of the question and you can almost guarantee at least a 3 for content. Do not neglect section 3 because I know people who aced the first two sections but didn't do too well on section 3. As a result, they did not get called for an interview.

**"The greatest enemy of knowledge is not ignorance; it is the illusion of knowledge – Stephen Hawking. Write an essay in which you address the following points: in science, how is the illusion of knowledge an enemy of knowledge? Can you argue that ignorance itself an enemy of knowledge? By what criteria could you assess the comparative impact of**

**these two, to determine which is the greater enemy of scientific knowledge?"**

Here is a typical essay question from section 3. You will get a choice so pick the one you are most comfortable with. Some of these questions can be a bit philosophical so keep that in mind. There is no right or wrong answer. As long as you can present valid arguments. Oh, and please do not make information up. Examiners do check these things. Your essay will be marked by 2 examiners. They will each assign a grade and the average will be taken. For example, if the two examiners give you a score of 2A and 4C. The final score would be the average which is 3B.

# Chapter Four: Personal Statement Tips

Your personal statement is a very important part of your application. I believe it's the silliest part because it tells you nothing interesting about the candidate and it's often written and edited by others. Don't let that put you off. You can still write a quality personal statement without paying a single penny. Universities will use your personal statement in different ways, but it is a chance to "sell yourself". It doesn't really include your academic achievements. It's all about you and why the university should call you for an interview. This is where you mention all your work experience and extra-curricular activities. The structure should be clear. The personal statement is 4000 characters over 47 lines. Let's take a look at how you should structure your personal statement.

## **Introduction**

This is the first thing the university will see when they read your personal statement. Please do not include cliché openers such as "ever since I was a little kid...". The introduction is the part you mention *why* you want to study medicine. Why do you want to become a doctor? What is your motivation? You will need to think about this deeply because it can make or break your application. I would recommend dedicating one well thought out paragraph about why you want to study medicine.

## **Work Experience/Volunteering**

This is arguably the most important part of your personal statement. It shows dedication and motivation to study medicine. Earlier, we mentioned *where* you can do your work experience. This is where it all comes into play. So, let's say you have completed three different work experience/volunteering opportunities. You take one of these and state what it was and what it involved (you can also mention how long you did it for to show dedication). You mention an example of something you witnessed or took part in. This could be a consultation between a doctor and patient, a handover meeting between members of the multi-disciplinary team (MDT) or a conversation you had with a patient. Keep it short and sweet. Don't make it look like you're narrating a story. Then you mention what you learned from this experience. This is the most crucial part. Med schools don't care if you watched live surgery or even performed the damn surgery yourself. They don't expect you to throw around medical vocabulary nor do they expect you to know how to perform procedures. They just want to know what you learnt from this experience. When I say 'what you learnt' I don't mean medical knowledge. I mean personal development. What do you now know about the MDT? What have you learnt about the reality of being a doctor? Have your communication skills improved? These are the things med schools want to see. After that's done, you move on to your next work experience and follow the same structure. I would recommend at least three different placements/volunteering opportunities and three different things you have developed.

## **Wider Reading/Exploration**

This is a chance for you to show how much extra reading or studying you have done. If you have read any interesting books you can mention that here and what you learnt from it. Please don't lie on your personal statement about anything. I know someone who mentioned how they read a book only to be interviewed by the author of that book (thank God he didn't lie but don't get caught out). This part shouldn't be too long and can be integrated with your extra-curricular activities.

## **Extra-curricular Activities**

This part simply mentions anything else you have taken part in. I was part of the UCL Target Medicine programme, so I mentioned that. It can be the Duke of Edinburgh award or anything of the sort. I would mention why you would be suitable as a student at this university. Do not mention universities by name as they all receive the same personal statement but mention what *you* can offer *them*. They don't want robots who study all day and nothing else. If you're interested in joining or starting up a society then mention that. If you are part of a sports team or have any interesting hobbies, then mention that. Show them you have a lot to offer as a student. This also shows that you can manage a busy schedule.

## **Conclusion**

The conclusion should be short and sweet. Literally two or three sentences will suffice. Just summarise why you are a good candidate and your motivation to study medicine.

I recommend **not paying** a company or a person to write or edit your personal statement. These people do not care about you – they care about money.

When it comes to editing your personal statement, I recommend having two people go over it. The first person should be a medical student or someone similar to see if the content is appropriate. The next person should be an

English teacher or someone similar to check over your spelling, grammar and sentence syntax. Having many people go over your statement can get confusing as it creates many different opinions.

**Under no circumstance should you plagiarise any part of your personal statement or you risk losing your chance to study medicine.**

# Chapter Five: Interview Tips

My favourite part. I love interviews. They're meant to be tense but for me they're just conversations. However, if you have made it this far into your application then congratulations! I have good news: the university wants you. They see you as a potential student. Now all you have to do is sell yourself and prove why they should give you an offer. We will first go through some general interview tips before going into the different types of interviews. We will then look at some common questions and how you can answer them.

## General Interview Tips

- Dress the part – no tracksuits or casual clothes. It is better to overdress than underdress. Go for a more formal/professional look. Although your outfit won't get you any extra marks, it will make a good first impression.

- Use personal examples – if it's possible, mention an example of a task you performed to demonstrate your capabilities.

- If you don't want to praise yourself and seem arrogant, mention how other people have praised you.

- Read Tomorrow's Doctors by the GMC. It will give you a better understanding of a doctor's role.

- Always mention the multi-disciplinary team whenever possible. Interviewers love this phrase for some reason but make sure what you say is meaningful. Again, try and use a personal example.

- Refer back to the four pillars of medical ethics: autonomy, beneficence, non-maleficence and justice.

- Do not waffle – make sure you answer the question.

- Make sure everything you have said in your personal statement is true because if you get asked about something and you lied about it then you know… you kinda screwed up.

- If you are asked an ethical question, mention both sides and do not immediately blurt out an answer. They want you to think deeply about it.

## **Traditional Panel Interview**

This kind of interview is the standard face to face interview. You will be asked questions from a variety of medical professionals for about 20-40 minutes. Be genuine and be confident. These people are experienced and can see it from a mile away when you are pretending to be something you are not. Do not rehearse answers. I've sat through a tonne of mock interviews and real interviews and I have never felt stressed or pressured. I never practised answers and I was always genuine. So here are some tips for the panel interview.

- Don't shake hands but smile. I know it sounds bad to not shake hands, but it can make the interview very awkward if not done correctly. I once had an interview where the table between us was so long that it was impossible to shake hands without walking across the room. Just smile instead and look pleased.

- Maintain eye contact with every single person on the panel equally – even if they didn't ask you the question. Make it look like you are speaking to all of them when you answer a question.

- Again, use personal examples whenever possible. Mention the MDT and four pillars whenever possible.

- Use examples from your work experience to demonstrate your skills if asked.

- Be yourself. Remember, these interviewers have done this for years and will see right through your act.

- Do not rehearse answers – they will notice it very easily.

- You cannot predict questions based off of what your friends had – don't bother with this.

- Research the medical school you are being interviewed at.

Ask your college if they can arrange mock interviews for students applying for medicine. This would give you a chance to practice and get used to the feeling. Again, I do not recommend paying for interview crash courses or anything like that. Save your money.

## **MMI**

Some universities use an MMI instead of a panel one. A multiple mini interview consists of 10 stations (can vary depending on the med school) with each station lasting approximately 10 minutes. One of these stations is often an acting station where you will have to break bad news to a professional actor pretending to be a character. Here are some tips for an MMI.

- Always answer the question. One of the stations may have more than one question so be sure to answer everything – use examples!

- If you mess up a station – don't worry! The stations are not linked, and the next interviewer will not be aware of your other stations so approach each station with a fresh mind.

- You don't need to put on an Oscar-worthy performance for the acting station. The main thing you want to do is show **empathy** and **good communication skills**. Offer an appropriate solution to the problem.

- If you finish a station early, don't start a conversation with the interviewer. They will ignore you (and think you're a weirdo).

- Some interviewers may put on a mean look to try and put you off. Just ignore that and answer the question. Maintain a casual smile.

- Some stations may have nothing got to do with medicine, but they test key skills. Be aware of this.

- If you need clarification – ask! Don't try to answer a question you do not completely understand.

- You may be given an ethical question. Remember to weigh up both sides before answering.

- I got asked a question about choosing between a med school offer and a job with a 40k starting salary and brand-new BMW. *Please* don't pick anything other than the med school offer. It may sound obvious but don't forget you are in an interview for *med school.* You can mention how you appreciate the job offer and how it may tempt others, but still kindly refuse it because you want to become a doctor.

- Another question I was asked was if I would sign-in for a friend on their behalf. It doesn't matter who it involves – follow the rules and don't sign-in for them.

# Chapter Six: Exam Preparation

You thought I'd just give you tips on getting into medical school? Nope. Now I'm going to teach you how to smash your exams. Following this method will guarantee you at least 3 A's and even A*'s if you're *really* dedicated. So, you've picked your A-Level subjects, completed the UCAT/BMAT and passed your interview. You now have an offer for medical school. Congratulations! But the real work begins now. All of this would have been for nothing if you do not meet the grade requirements on results day. If I'm completely honest, A-Levels aren't that difficult. If you put in the time and effort, you will see results. This guide will assume you are studying biology, chemistry and maths.

## **AS Level**

Your first year of college will be tough – well at least the first few weeks or months will be. It is quite the leap from GCSEs, but it is still manageable. You may even see some E or U grades initially which is heart-breaking but don't worry. In my first ever college assessment I got D, E, U and U for my subjects. At the end of the two years, I had only A's and A*'s. Was it because I went from being dumb to clever? No. It was because I went from being lazy to hard working. I went from playing PlayStation 4 and training all day to revising for a solid number of hours every day. You want at least 3 A grades at the end of your first year. This will give you at least 3 As for your predicted grades. You'll want at least one A* prediction just to boost your application but the more the better. This may sound harsh but if you do not have at least 3 A grades predicted, you have an *extremely* low chance of being called for an interview – basically impossible unless it includes a foundation year. Consider taking a gap year if that is the case. The main thing for this year: secure at least 3 As and get an A*AA prediction or better (especially if you are applying to Oxbridge). The technique to get the grades will be explained below.

## **A2**

You thought the jump from GCSEs to AS was bad? The jump from AS to A2 is terrifying at first. However, by now you should have a solid routine and by using the method I'm about to mention, you should find it easy.

### **Biology**

There is a reason why biology has a lower grade boundary than most subjects – the exam is very picky. You will need to mention keywords in order to secure marks. Here is how I got an A* in A-Level biology. First, you will need to learn the content. I finished learning the entire specification by myself in the summer before A2 started. By the time the new academic year began, all I needed was practice and I would have been ready for the exam in December. Is it because I was a nerdy guy with nothing better to do (kind of)? No, it was because I wanted to succeed and outwork everyone else. Don't get me wrong, I still had a life. I only did a maximum of three hours a day during the summer. I still kept all of my hobbies and had a blast. If you want to beat everyone, you have to be prepared to do things they aren't doing. Your teachers will probably advise against what I did but then again, this method is not for everyone. So, the way I finished all of the content in summer was using the AQA specification, a CGP revision guide and YouTube videos. Go through the specification to see what topic you should learn and make short notes as you go along (you do not need to use fancy colours and glitter pens to make notes in case some of you didn't know *cough*). Making notes isn't extremely important as you can use the CGP book as your notes. Work smarter, not harder! SnapRevise has really good videos on biology so I would watch some of their free videos on YouTube. Draw diagrams for difficult concepts such as action potentials or whatever you find difficult. Remember, if you find anything difficult to understand, wait until college starts and ask your teacher. Your teachers are there to help you. Don't think you're a badass who doesn't need a teacher because you're doing it by yourself. There were many times I asked my biology teacher (shout-out Mrs O. Markoulides the G.O.A.T) for help after school and she kindly helped me out. Once you have finished the specification the fun begins. Your mission, should you choose to accept it, will be to finish every single past paper (for your exam board) in existence before the actual A2 exams. You will have 3 papers at the end of the year, and you will want to ace all 3 of them. I highly recommend physicsandmathstutor.com for past papers. Make a list of all of them (including the old specification) and tick them off as you complete them. Don't rush to finish them all. And do not burn yourself out or you will regret it. Space out the days you do an exam paper and only around February or March time should you be doing one biology past paper a day. I cannot emphasise enough how important it is to not burn out. This method can be tiring so get proper rest. At around late April time, you should aim to hit your peak and be demolishing 4 past papers a day (one for biology, one for chemistry and two for maths) or 5 if you do 4 subjects. At first, when you do past papers you will get a lot of things wrong. Complete the paper, mark with a green or red pen and in a separate notebook, make a note of what you got wrong along with the correction (this notebook will help you a lot when exam time comes). You will struggle a lot... I mean a lot. Maybe getting less than 40% of the marks. However, the more papers you do, the easier it gets. At my peak, I was finishing most past papers in an hour and securing 85%+. Once you finish all of the past papers, you should move onto another exam board. I finished all the AQA papers and started Edexcel papers. I didn't do all of the Edexcel ones and I did leave the most recent AQA papers to do when my actual exams were closer. By now, you should have a little notebook (for every subject) with tonnes of mistakes you made whilst doing past papers. A few days before your actual exam keep going over this book and drill into your head the silly mistakes you made. Avoid these during the exam. The day of your exam has come. Remain calm and try to avoid hanging out with other people – this will only stress you. I personally never touch any revision on the day of an exam. Your two years of hard work and your med school offer all comes down to this. After hours of practice, the exam will honestly feel like a revision session. Read the question properly and do what you do best! If you followed this guide closely you will get an A at least.

## **Chemistry**

The guide for chemistry is honestly the same but with a few changes. I didn't finish the chemistry specification until December but don't focus too much on rushing to finish. It's about learning the new information and not speed running through the syllabus. I would say finishing the syllabus for all of your subjects before the March is solid. Follow the guide for biology but instead of the CGP guide etc. Use a website called chemrevise.org. You don't even need to make your own notes for chemistry because chemrevise has amazing ones that you can print out and use. Chemrevise along with Allery Chemistry on YouTube will give you a solid understanding of chemistry. All that's left is to practice. Again, the same way you did for biology. Make a list of all the papers and do them all (papers can be found on physicsandmathstutor.com). They will get easier the more you do. Have a little notebook to write down all of your mistakes and go through it regularly. There's not much else to say other than stay consistent but don't burn out. Once you finish your exam board, move onto another exam board or even practice some questions by topic if you are weak in a particular topic.

### Mathematics

I loved maths up until A-Levels. In fact, I did my maths GCSE in year 10 (and got an A*). However, when I reached my first year of A-Levels, I was lost. Not doing any pure maths in year 11 hurt my maths knowledge. I had forgotten the most basic things such as factorising quadratics and basic algebra. This was evident after I saw my results for my first maths A-Level assessment. I got 3/40. No, that's not a typo. I actually did get THREE out of FORTY – one of the lowest in my year group. But now I'm in med school. So why am I telling you all this? Because the first few weeks of A-Levels *will* be hard, but you *will* adapt. The new specification doesn't allow you to pick between statistics and mechanics – you have to do both. Do not fret! I will teach you how to succeed in maths. In my opinion, maths is easier to learn at home than biology and chemistry. Your maths teacher may disagree with me and that's fine. Like I said, this method is not for everyone but those who use it well will succeed. Aim to finish the syllabus before January. You do not need to spend a single penny on maths textbooks because maths is mainly application and not much memorising. The best resource is YouTube. My favourite channel was Exam Solutions. Use the Edexcel (or your exam board) specification and go through the topics on his YouTube channel. He will explain the topic to you and answer a question, showing you how it's done. All of his videos will include some questions for you to try while you pause the video – do these! You cannot learn maths by watching videos and expecting to learn. You will only become good at maths after you have done hundreds of practice questions. Once you feel like you have understood the concept, move onto questions by topic. An abundance of these can be found on physicsandmathstutor.com. Practice as many questions you can on each topic until you feel like you can do these in your sleep. Once you feel confident, have a go at a full exam paper. Since the specification is new, I would recommend using old spec papers and timing yourself. Do one or two new spec papers but save the majority of them for later. Remember to make a note of all the mistakes you make in your little notebook. The more papers you do the easier and quicker it gets. At my peak, I was finishing an entire paper in less than 45 minutes. I know a guy who used to finish the paper TWICE during the actual exam and used both of his attempts to compare his answers (he used to almost always get full marks in every exam). Now here's the important part: you also have your statistics and mechanics to worry about. Do the exact same for these. However, once you reach March/April time, you should be doing two maths papers a day. One for pure maths and one for statistics and mechanics. Combine this with your other subjects and you should be doing a minimum of four papers a day. It might seem like a lot, but you'll eventually get more efficient at completing them.

## **My A-Levels Experience**

So, I kept mentioning how I was 'at my peak', right? Well, let me explain what this consisted of and how my day went. All of this was from March onwards. I was doing 4 past papers a day. One for biology, one for chemistry, one for pure maths and one for applied maths (statistics). I would attend college as normal. I would take part in class like a normal student. Sometimes, during chemistry class, my teacher (shout-out Mr J. Parslow) would let me do a past paper in class. I used this opportunity to get one of my four past papers out of the way. I normally had two private study sessions every day, so I did one past paper per session. By the time school was finished, I had already completed three out of four past papers. See how simple it looks now? I stayed back in the library and finished my last paper for the day before 4:30 pm. I got home before 5 pm and had all the free time in the world to do whatever I liked. At first, you might have thought I was working too hard. However, my methodology is always to work smart and not hard. I do not ever look at how long I revise for. Outside of college, I never revised for more than 2 hours except on weekends. Instead, I focus on completing my daily dose of revision. Whether I have an amazing day and finish it all in two hours or I procrastinate and take six hours, it must be done before the next day. It doesn't matter whether it's done in the morning or night, in college or at home, on the floor or hanging from my ceiling, it gets done. To be honest, I could have done even better in my A-Level exams if I did more work. However, I wanted to have fun and I was never too fussed about having the highest grades in the class. I balanced my revision with my other interests such as martial arts, gaming, art and many others. I never saw myself as the smartest kid in the class nor did I ever put myself down. Grades are not a reflection of your intelligence; they are a reflection of your effort. Surround yourself with hard workers and it will motivate and inspire you. I looked up to two of my friends who were a year older than me and a lot of the advice I am giving you now is the advice they gave me.

I have seen people mess around in college and end up in tears on results day. I never wanted that to be me. Take your education seriously and I promise you will not regret it when you make it into med school.

**Disclaimer: the method highlighted above may not be suitable for everyone. Finishing an A-Level syllabus by yourself is not easy so you *can* go through it with your college instead. However, the part about completing all of the past exam papers is a must.**

# PART II: From Med Student to Doctor

In part one, we looked at the journey from college to med school. In part two, we will focus on med school itself, particularly the first year. The transition from college to university is tough. You are exposed to a new level of freedom when it comes to studying. No one will be there to hold your hand or tell you what to do. There are no parents' evenings or detentions.

We will first take a look at some of the realities of studying medicine before I share some advice on how to survive and make the most of your first year.

# Chapter Seven: The Reality of Med School

Med school is not easy at all. At first, I did struggle quite a bit. Everything was just so different from what I was used to. I didn't know anyone; it was a new location and the structure of the learning was so different. The first thing you should know is that your day will typically start at 9 am and finish at 5 pm. On Wednesdays you will finish earlier for sports etc. You may have anatomy sessions where you learn about the human body…using a real human body…but a dead one. Some people tend to freak out a little while others faint and vomit. You'll probably get used to dissection room. Don't be afraid to ask to sit down if you feel a little light-headed. There will be a tonne of content to learn. Med school doesn't ease you in nice and slowly. You head straight into a "recap" of A-Level biology but in a much more detailed way. Each med school is different in the way they teach but you will start by learning pre-clinical knowledge in the first few years.

Whilst the majority of med students are nice, some can be slithery snakes. They will *not* hesitate to leave you in the dust if it benefits them – but this is rare. Sure, some med students will walk around with a stethoscope around their neck thinking they're doctors already, but just ignore them.

You are expected to behave differently to other students. You are a med student and a future doctor therefore you will have a lot of responsibility in the way you carry yourself. If you have social media, be careful what you say. Don't get involved in any crime or do anything stupid like avoiding a train fare. You may also come across some party animals who may be into illegal drugs – stay away from them. If you do get into any legal trouble, inform your med school. They will guide you through what you need to do. You will get into trouble for things like breaching confidentiality, pretending to be a doctor or performing unconsented examinations.

You may find yourself behind in your studies and overwhelmed. This is normal. For many students, med school is a game of catching up. This isn't like college where you can finish the syllabus by yourself (I wish).

You will soon be required to attend placements. At first, you will feel like you're just getting in the way. As you progress through the years, you will still feel the same, but you will be more involved with patients and their treatment.

# Chapter Eight: Survive Your First Year

Right, this is the part where I give you some advice on how to make the most of your first year. Hold on tight and don't be afraid to have fun.

- Don't buy any textbooks unless your university tells you to.

- Ignore people who say "first year doesn't matter" because it does. It will build the foundation that you need for the following year. Always try your best!

- You don't need a huge friendship group but do make friends with some of the older medics. They will have valuable advice (and their notes) to share with you.

- Attend lectures if you can but if you are like me and you cannot learn from being inside the lecture theatre then don't go – unless they require you to sign in!

- During the fresher's fair, join every society and get as much free stuff as you can. Trust me, there you may come across some cool freebies.

- You may not need a stethoscope during your first year so check with your university.

- Stay on top of your lectures. The last thing you want is to be 20 lectures behind with an exam coming up.

- You *can* work part-time during med school but make sure it doesn't affect your studies.

- Don't compare yourself to your peers. You may or may not be the top of your class anymore but just give it your best shot.

- Use your first few weeks of med school to determine your study method early on. This could be writing notes, flashcards or watching lectures. I highly recommend using active recall and spaced repetition.

- Have some hobbies or activities you enjoy outside of med school

- Seek help from student support if you are struggling with anything. Finance, mental health, studies or anything else. They are there to help *you*.

## *About the Author*

*I'm supposed to write this part in third person, right? Screw that. My name is Ahmed Ali. I am a 3$^{rd}$-year medical student studying in London.*

*I was born and raised in East London where I still live. Growing up, I always changed my career aspirations. I wanted to become a footballer, then a teacher, then an MMA fighter, then an accountant, then an engineer and finally a doctor. I have an interest in general practice and surgery. However, I would love to have my own GP practice in the area that I grew up. I'd also love to start my own business one day.*

*I didn't grow up in a rich family, but I always made the most of what I had and the opportunities I was given. I was sick of seeing aspiring medics get charged hundreds for medical "experience" and training. I decided to write this short book and make it easily accessible for all. Medicine should not be for the rich only. Those who have what it takes to be the next generation of doctors should be given the chance to study medicine.*

*Let's talk a bit about my education. I went to a normal primary school in East London and a boys' secondary school. I picked up 10 GCSEs which were not the greatest but just slightly above average. I went on to study maths, biology, chemistry and economics at A-Level but dropped economics after the first year. My final grades were A\*AAa. I have always been an independent person when it comes to studying, often finding myself going ahead of everyone else. This has helped me rely on others less and not be spoon-fed information.*

*I have many hobbies such as martial arts, callisthenics, art and DIY. I have kept all of these hobbies throughout my journey to med school and even in med school. I always believe in working smart and getting the job done.*

*Money, fame and wealth means nothing to me. Helping others and leaving behind a legacy has always been my idea of success.*

*Go against all the odds and go fulfil your destiny.*

Printed in Great Britain
by Amazon